90-DAY NO EQUIPMENT WORKOUT PLAN

EASY TO FOLLOW FULL BODY EVERYDAY WORKOUT PLANS FOR ALL AGES AT HOME

ALEX FITZENSTEIN

TABLE OF CONTENT

- Lower Body Exercises
- Core Strengthening Workouts

Conclusion

Introduction

This is the **"90-Day No Equipment Workout Plan: Easy to Follow Full Body Everyday Workout Plans for All Ages at Home."** With the aid of this book, you may start a fitness adventure that will change your life without having to pay for a fancy gym membership or costly equipment. This training regimen, which emphasises simplicity and practicality, is appropriate for people of all ages and fitness levels and can be done comfortably in the comfort of your own home.

Let me start by telling you about me and how this workout routine came to be. I was in a scenario a few years ago that most of us can identify with. The stresses of daily life, a sedentary lifestyle, and a hectic schedule had all taken a toll on my health and wellbeing. I realised that something had to change, but I also realised that going to the gym on a daily basis might not be an option.

That's how I first learned about the idea of at-home workouts. Though I was initially dubious, I began experimenting with various regimens and eventually discovered the effectiveness of bodyweight exercises and the amazing outcomes they could provide. What began as a dedication to a 90-day fitness regimen evolved into a way of life shift. Along with getting fitter and more energised, my general health also seemed to have significantly improved.

The efficacy of at-home workouts is demonstrated by the 90-Day No Equipment Workout Plan included in this book. It's proof that getting in shape doesn't require an ostentatious gym or pricey equipment. All you need is the will to get started, the perseverance to keep going, and the understanding of how to complete full-body exercises.

You will find a thorough, step-by-step approach to a full-body exercise programme in this book.

The exercises are thoughtfully crafted to be easy to perform and don't call for any specialised gear. These exercises can be customised to meet your needs, regardless of your degree of experience or desire to maintain and improve your present fitness.

It's time to start your own fitness adventure now that we have outlined the main points of this book. Prepare to enjoy the comforts of home training, along with the mental and physical advantages that come with consistent exercise. Along with assisting you in reaching your fitness objectives, this exercise programme will give you the self-assurance that you can manage your health and wellbeing.

Now let's begin this amazing 90-day journey to a happier, fitter, and healthier version of ourselves. Never forget that you have the ability to change, and this book is here to support you every step of the way. Prepare to be amazed by the transformational power of at-home workouts without any equipment!

Day 1-30 Beginner Workouts

- **Day 1-2 Full Body Warm-Up**

Start with a mild warm-up for the entire body that incorporates simple aerobic exercises like jumping jacks or stationary running. To prepare your muscles and raise your heart rate, give each workout five to ten minutes of effort.

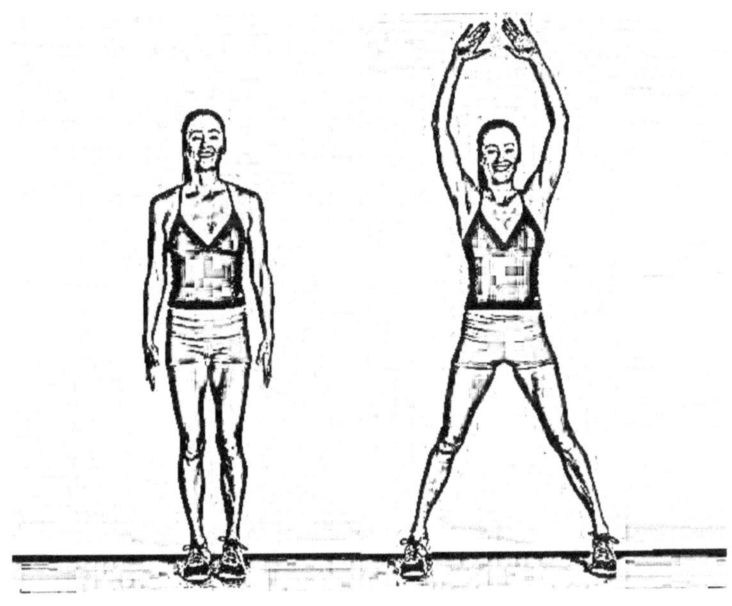

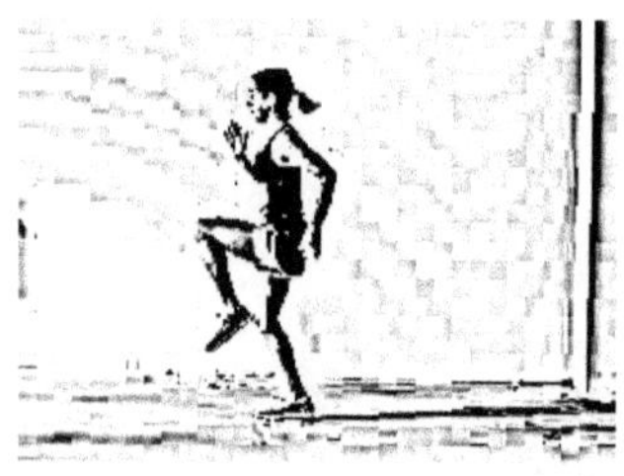

- **Day 3-4 Core and Balance**

Planks: Hold the position for 20–30 seconds, extending the duration a little bit each time.

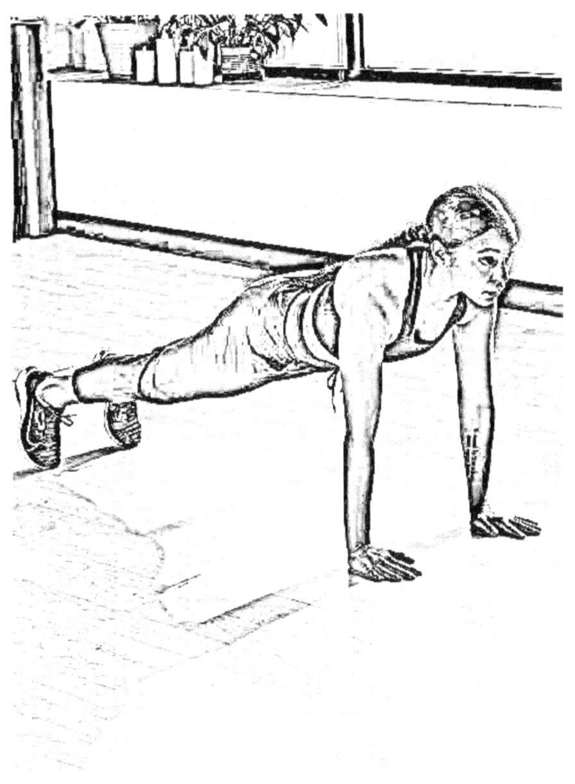

Glute Bridges: Raise your hips and tense your glutes while lying on your back with your knees bent. Do 12–15 reps in 3 sets.

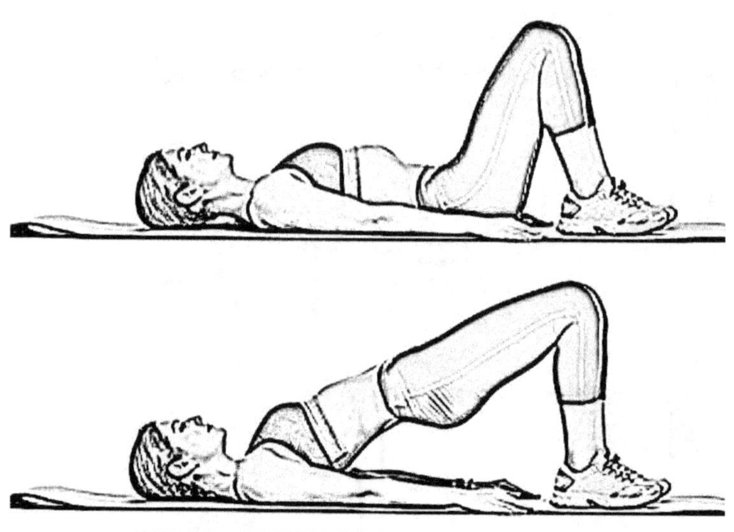

Cardio Workout: Do a 20–30 minute aerobic workout, such as jogging, cycling, or brisk walking. Keep a steady but challenging pace for yourself.

Push-ups: As you advance, increase the number of sets and repetitions. Begin with two sets of five to seven push-ups.

Tricep dips: Perform two sets of 10–12 repetitions on a stable surface (such as a chair).

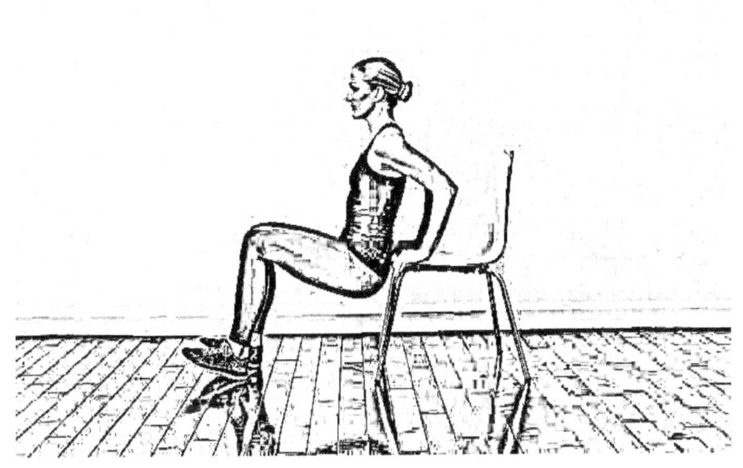

- **Day 9-10 Lower Body Focus**

Bodyweight Squats: Concentrate on your form and start with two sets of ten to twelve squats.

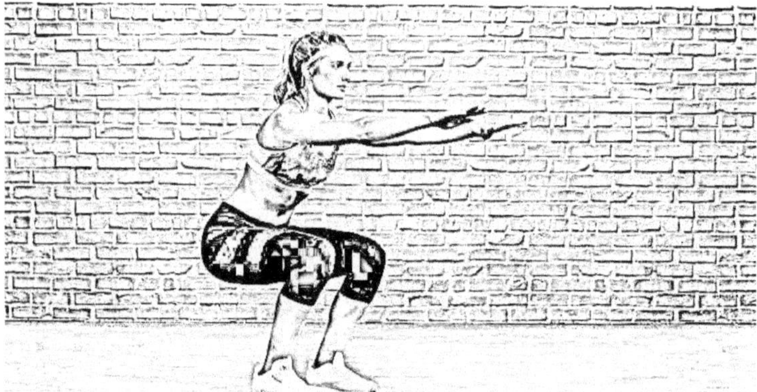

Lunges: Do ten to twelve lunges per leg in two sets.

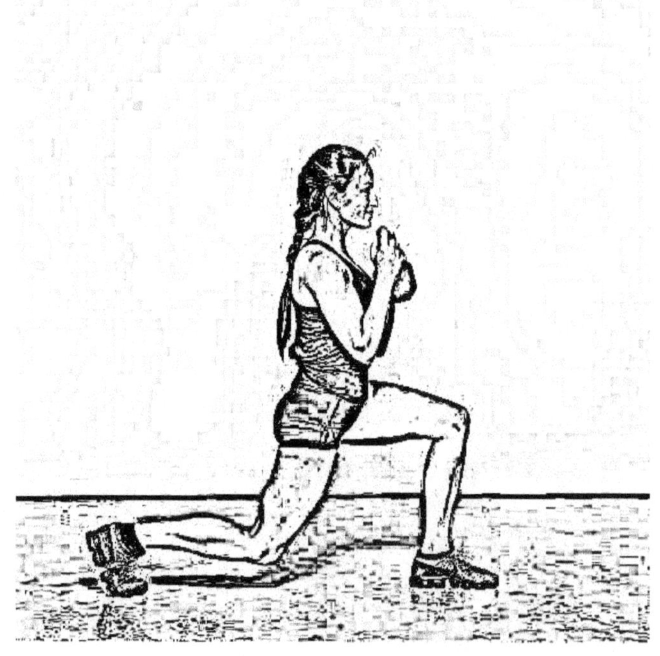

During this time, be sure to pay attention to your body and perform each exercise with correct form. If you've never exercised before, the goal of the first 10 days is to get comfortable with the movements and create a regular habit. Your strength and endurance will grow as you go along, getting you ready for the harder parts of the 90-day plan. For best effects, remember to stay hydrated, eat healthily, and get enough sleep.

Well done on finishing the first ten days of your 90-day fitness programme without using any equipment! Now that you've established the foundation, it's time to intensify your workout and carry on with your fitness adventure. We'll concentrate on increasing strength, enhancing endurance, and adding some diversity to your exercise regimen during days 11 through 20.

- **Day 11-12 Full Body Strength**

Push-Ups: Increase to three sets of eight to ten push-ups.

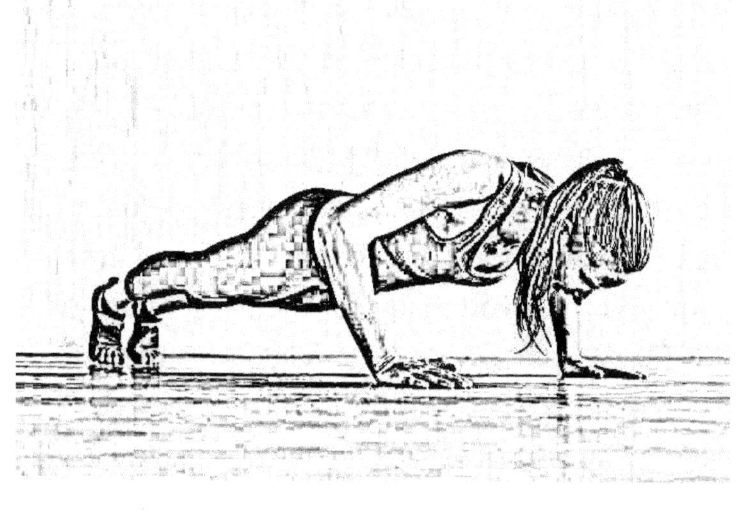

Bodyweight Squats: Complete three sets of
12–15 bodyweight squats.

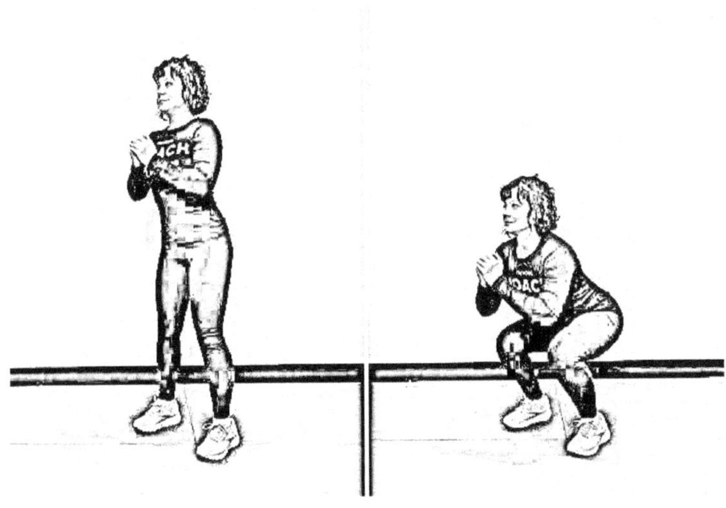

- **Day 13-14 Cardio and Endurance**

Cardio Workout: Increase the duration of your workout to 30 to 40 minutes while keeping a fast-paced yet manageable intensity.

Incorporate training intervals: Switch between shorter, lower-intensity recovery intervals and longer, higher-intensity bursts (such as sprinting or faster-paced activity).

Planks: For planks, aim for three sets of thirty to forty seconds.

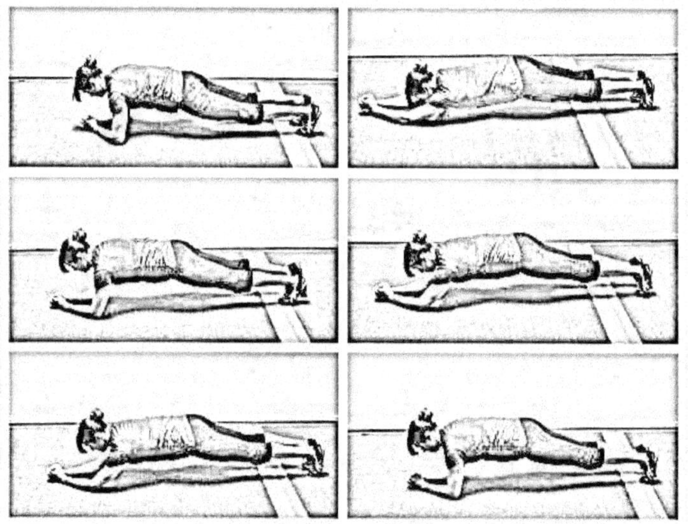

Russian Twists: While seated on the floor, slant your shoulders back a little, then twist your body such that each side touches the floor. Do 12–15 repetitions per side in 3 sets.

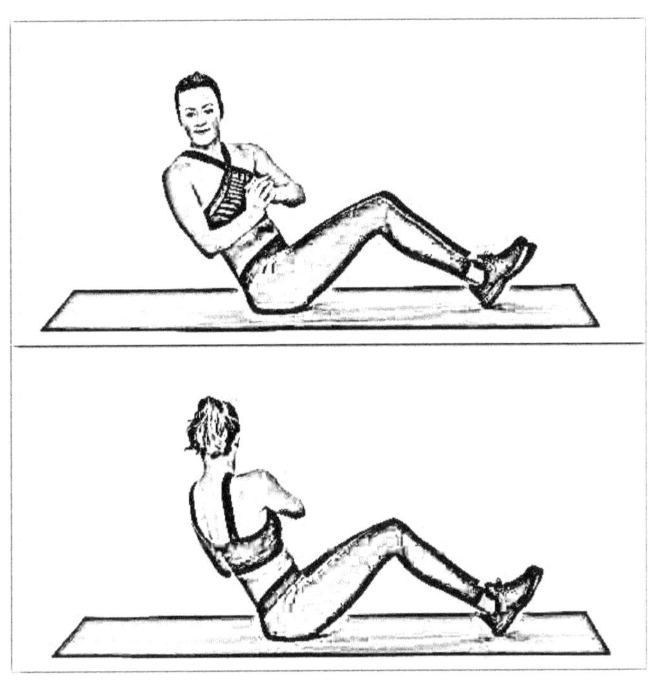

Push-ups: Complete three sets of ten to twelve push-ups.

Tricep dips: Try three sets of 12–15 repetitions for the tricep dips.

Diamond Push-Ups: Form a diamond shape with your hands close together, then perform two sets of 6–8 repetitions.

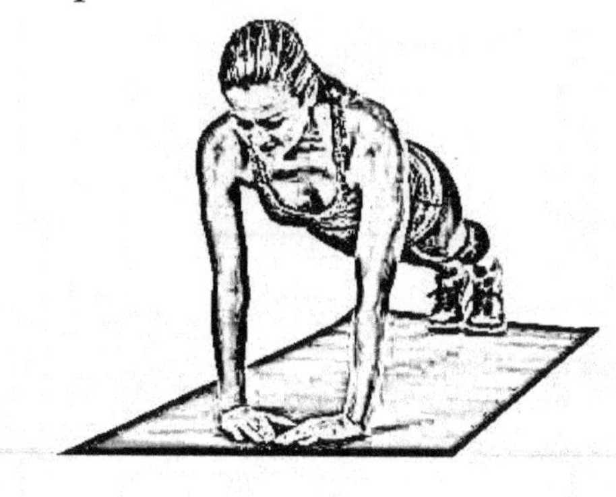

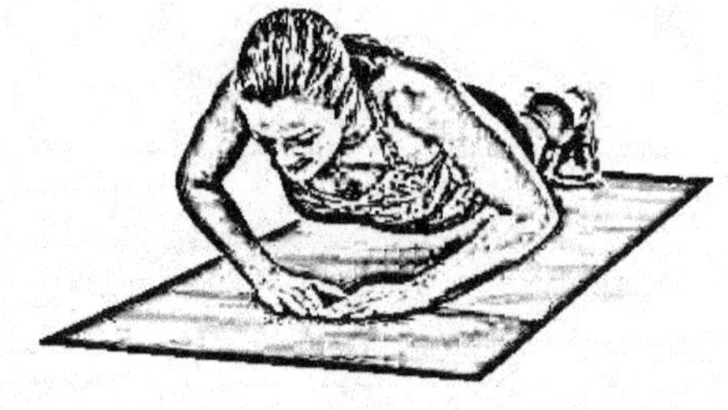

- **Day 19-20 Lower Body Focus**

Bodyweight squats: Perform three sets of 15 to 20 bodyweight squats.

Lunges: Increase to 12–15 lunges per leg in three sets.

Calf Raises: To strengthen your calves, elevate your heels while standing on a step or platform. Do 3 sets of 15–20 repetitions.

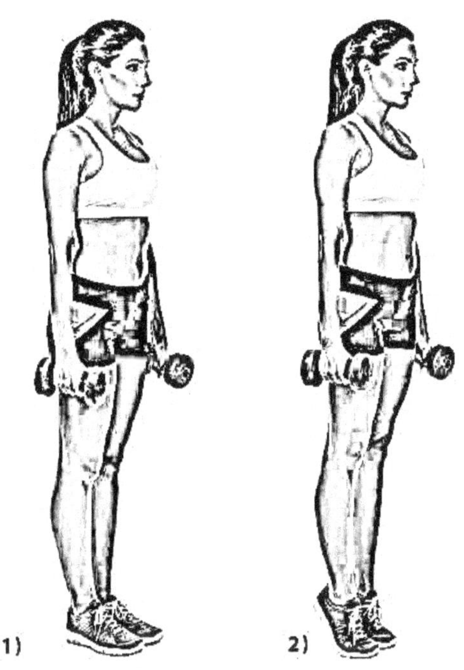

Your strength and endurance will start to improve throughout this phase. Your limits will be pushed by adding increasingly difficult workouts and doing longer cardio sessions. Recall to breathe regularly, keep yourself hydrated, and maintain correct form. You'll be ready for the next stages of the training programme when your body adjusts to the increased workload. Remain dedicated and keep moving forward with your fitness journey.

- **Day 21-22 Full Body Strength and Core**

Push-Ups: Perform 3 sets of 10–12 repetitions.

Bodyweight squats: Perform three sets of fifteen to twenty bodyweight squats.

Planks: Up to three sets of 40–50 seconds for the planks.
Start with two sets of 20–25 repetitions each leg for mountain climbers.

- **Day 23-24 Cardio and Endurance**

Cardio workout: Increase the duration of your cardio workout to 40–50 minutes.

If you can work out on an incline or a hill, including such into your routine.

For an additional challenge, stick to your interval training regimen.

- **Day 25-26 Upper Body and Core Focus**

Diamond Push Ups: Add three sets of eight to ten repetitions for the diamond push-up.

Tricep dips: Perform 3 sets of 12–15 repetitions.

Russian Twists: 3 sets of 15–20 repetitions on each side.

Plank Rotations: On both sides, rotate your torso until your hips are in contact with the floor. Do 10–12 repetitions per side in two sets.

- **Day 27-28 Lower Body Strength and Balance**

Bodyweight squats: Complete three sets of 20–25 bodyweight squats.

Lunges: Increase to three sets of fifteen to twenty lunges each leg.

Single-Leg Glute Bridges: Raise your hips and one leg while lying on your back. Do 12–15 reps in two sets for each leg.

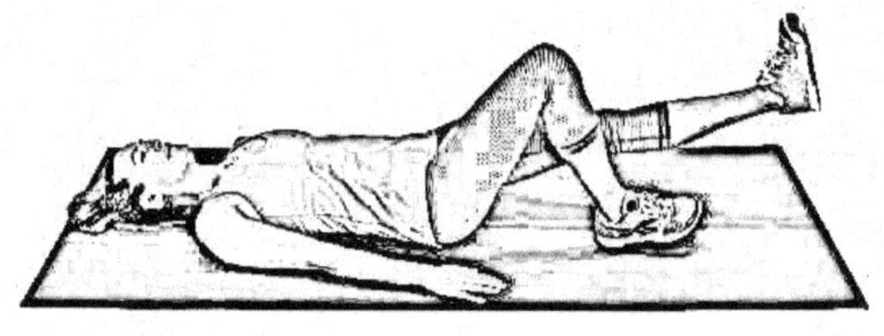

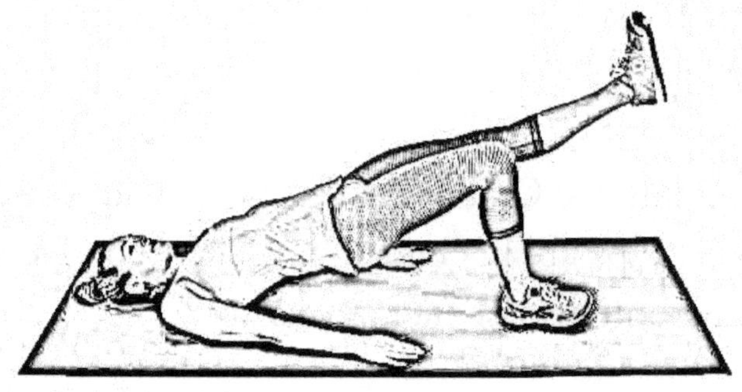

- **Day 29-30 Full Body Circuit**

For a full-body circuit workout, mix and match exercises from earlier in the week.
Take a 15-second break after every 30 seconds of exercise.
Finish the circuit's three rounds.

Over the course of these 30 days, push yourself while adhering to correct form and technique. You'll push yourself to the limit and make great strides in strength, endurance, and general fitness with the longer cardio workouts and more difficult exercises. Remain concentrated, have an optimistic outlook, and never forget that the secret to achieving your fitness objectives is consistency. You're going to be a better, stronger version of yourself soon!

Progress Tracking

One of the most important parts of your 90-day no-equipment workout programme is tracking your progress. It not only keeps you motivated but also enables you to decide on changes to your routine with knowledge. Here's how to monitor your development efficiently:

1. Keep a Workout notebook: One of the easiest and most efficient ways to monitor your progress is to keep a workout notebook. Keep track of the exercises, sets, repetitions, and any performance comments you have for each workout. You can

also record your feelings and any difficulties you encountered during the exercise.

2. Take Regular Pictures: Prior to starting your ninety-day adventure, take pictures of yourself in well-lit settings and from different perspectives. Every ten days, or at the conclusion of each phase of the training schedule, repeat this process. By comparing these pictures throughout time, you can create a visual record of your development.

3. Track Measurements: Take measurements of your arms, legs, waist, hips, and chest, among other important body parts. Perform this at the start of your adventure and at the conclusion of every stage (days 10, 20, 30, etc.). Measurement changes may serve as a reliable indicator of your development.

4. Keep an eye on Your Weight and Body Composition: Although weight might be a useful indicator, you shouldn't rely solely on it. Track your weight consistently at the same time of day

(e.g., morning) using a bathroom scale. But take into account other aspects as well, such as body fat percentage, since muscular growth can counteract fat loss, rendering the scale an unreliable indicator of development.

5. Assess Strength and Endurance: Document the progress you've made in terms of your strength and endurance. Keep track of how many push-ups, squats, or other exercises you can complete in a given set. Gradual increases should be seen over time.

6. Listen to Your Body: Observe your post-workout and during-workout sensations. It's an indication of growth if you're feeling more capable, resilient, and strong. On the other hand, it could be time to reevaluate your regimen if you continue to endure pain or exhaustion.

7. Establish and Modify Objectives: Review your goals at the start of each phase (days 1, 11, 21, etc.) and make new ones. These can include particular fitness benchmarks, such hitting a goal

number of reps in an exercise or jogging a specific distance in a set amount of time. Modify your objectives to reflect your desires and progress.

8. Celebrate Your Success: Remember to give yourself a pat on the back for all of your small victories. Reaching your objectives, no matter how tiny, and finishing each phase are accomplishments that should be acknowledged. To keep oneself motivated, give yourself a worthwhile reward.

Not only does it help you stay motivated, but it also enables you to make well-informed decisions when it comes to modifying your exercise regimen. Monitoring your progress is crucial, regardless of whether you're changing your diet or the level of your workouts. Over the course of your 90-day workout plan, you'll see changes with dedication and consistency, even though growth isn't always linear.

Day 31-60 Intermediate Workouts

- **Day 31-32 Full Body Strength and Endurance**

Push-Ups: Do four sets of twelve to fifteen push-ups.

Bodyweight Squats: Perform four sets of fifteen to twenty squats.

Planks: Go up to four 45–60 second sets.

Mountain Climbers: Do three sets of 25–30 repetitions per leg for mountain climbers.

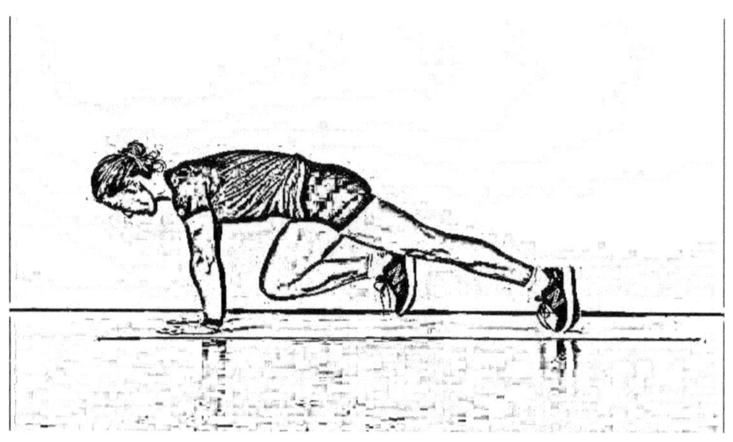

- **Day 33-34 Cardio and High-Intensity Interval Training (HIIT)**

Cardio Workout: Increase the duration of your cardio workout to 50–60 minutes.

Introduce HIIT: 30-second burpees or other high-intensity workouts should be alternated with 60 seconds of low-intensity recuperation.

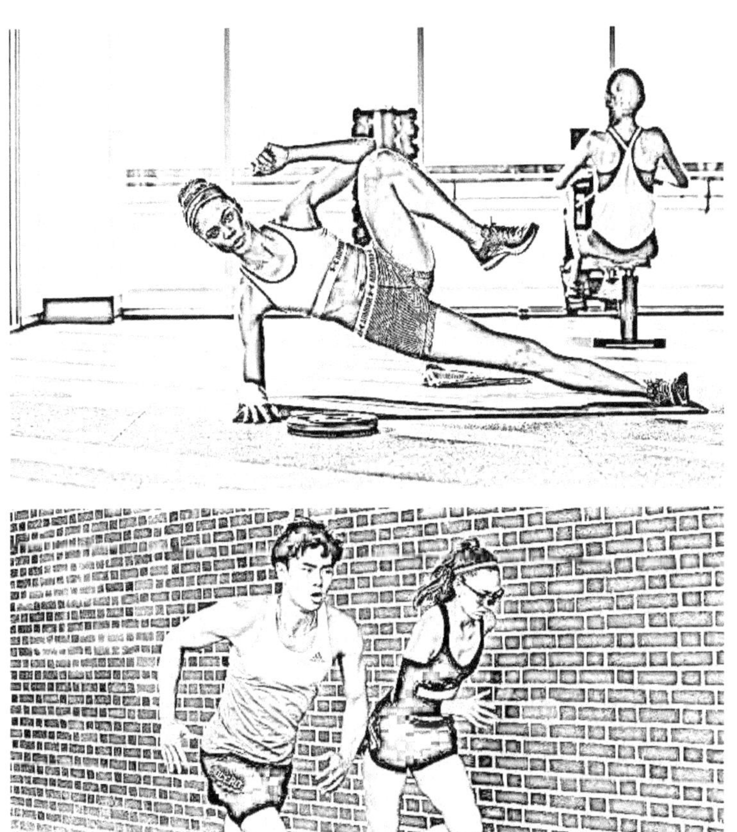

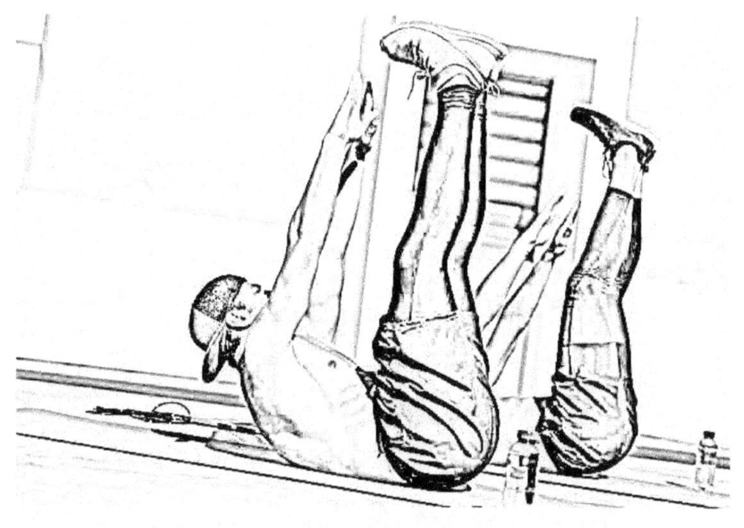

- **Day 35-36 Upper Body Strength and Core**

Diamond Push-Ups: 4 sets of 10–12 repetitions is the goal for diamond push-ups.

Tricep dip: Perform 4 sets of 15–20 repetitions for the tricep dip.

Russian twists: Increase to 4 sets of 20–25 repetitions per side for Russian twists.

Plank Rotations: Rotate your body in a plank posture for three sets of fifteen to twenty reps on each side.

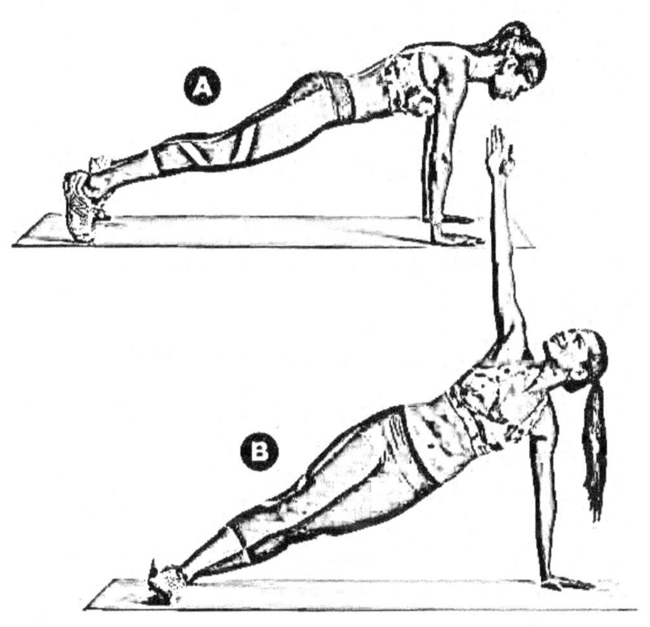

- **Day 37-38 Lower Body Strength and Balance**

Bodyweight squats: Perform four sets of twenty to twenty-five bodyweight squats.

Lunges: Perform four sets of fifteen to twenty lunges per leg.

Single-Leg Glute Bridges: For Single-Leg Glute Bridges, perform three sets of 15–20 repetitions per leg.

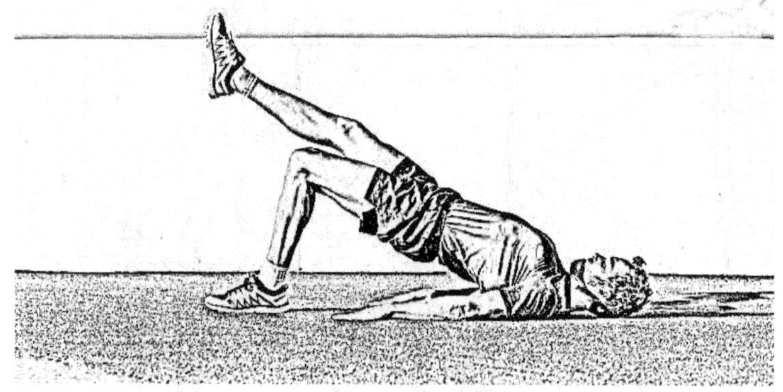

- **Day 39-40 Full Body Circuit and Progress Assessment**

Full Body Circuit: Incorporate a range of workouts from earlier days into a circuit training regimen.

Take a 15-second break after every 30 seconds of exercise.

Complete the circuit's four rounds.

Conduct a progress assessment following Day 40: Review your strength/endurance levels, measurements, and pictures to see how far you've progressed.

You'll be pushing yourself even harder throughout this phase. You may maintain your gains in strength, endurance, and fat reduction by upping the intensity of your workouts and implementing HIIT. Recall to breathe regularly, keep your form correct, and make sure you're getting enough nourishment and water. These ten days will be crucial to your path towards achieving your fitness goals, and you're well on your way. Maintain a strong sense of motivation and your dedication to success!

- **Day 41-42 Full Body Strength and Core**

Push-Ups: Do four sets of fifteen to eighteen push-ups.

Bodyweight Squats: Perform four sets of twenty to twenty-five squats.

Planks: Increase to 4 sets of 60–75 seconds for the planks.

Russian twists: Target four sets of 25–30 repetitions per side for Russian twists.

- **Day 43-44 Cardio and High Intensity Interval Training**

Cardio workout: Increase the duration of your cardio workout to 60–70 minutes.

HIIT Session: Use longer, more intense HIIT intervals. For example, 45 seconds of vigorous activity and 30 seconds of low-intensity recovery could be used.

- **Day 45-46**

Diamond Push-Ups: Perform 4 sets of 12–15 repetitions.

Tricep dip: Do four sets of 20–25 repetitions for the tricep dip.

Plank rotations: Increase to 4 sets of 20–25 repetitions per side for plank rotations.

Bicycle crunches: While lying on your back, cycle your legs till your elbow reaches the knee on the other side. Perform three sets of fifteen to twenty reps on each side.

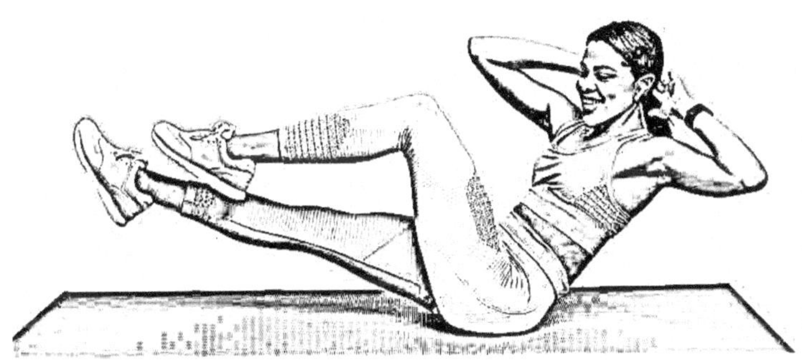

- Day 47-48

Bodyweight squats: Perform four sets of 25–30 bodyweight squats.

Lunges: Increase the number of lunges to four sets, 20–25 per leg.

Single-Leg Glute Bridges: For the single-leg glute bridges, perform three sets of 20–25 repetitions per leg.

Calf raises: Increase to 4 sets of 20–25 repetitions for the calf raises.

- **Day 49-50**

Whole Body Circuit: Mix and match workouts from earlier in the week to create a demanding circuit.

Take a 15-second break after every 30 seconds of exercise.

Complete the circuit's four rounds.

After Day 50, evaluate your progress by looking at your measurements, pictures, and strength/endurance levels to see how far you've come.

- Day 51-52

Push-Ups: Continue with 4 sets of 15-18 reps.

Bodyweight Squats: Perform 4 sets of 25-30 squats.

Planks: Increase to 4 sets of 75-90 seconds.

Mountain Climbers: Aim for 4 sets of 30-35 reps per leg.

- Day 53-54

Cardio workout: Increase the duration of your cardio workout to 70–80 minutes.

HIIT Session: Set a higher bar for yourself by completing longer, high-intensity intervals, like 60 seconds of vigorous exercise and 45 seconds of restorative low-intensity activity.

- **Day 55-56**

Diamond Push-Ups: Perform 4 sets of 15–18 repetitions.

Tricep dips: 4 sets of 25–30 repetitions.

Russian twists: Increase to 4 sets of 30–35 repetitions per side for Russian twists.

Plant rotation: Attempt four sets of 25–30 repetitions per side for plank rotations.

- **Day 57-58**

Bodyweight Squats: Perform four sets of thirty to thirty-five squats.

Lunges: Do 25–30 lunges per leg in 4 sets.

Glute Bridges on One Leg: Increase to Four Sets, 25–30 Reps Per Leg.

Calf Raises: Perform 4 sets of 25–30 repetitions.

- Day 59-60

Full Body Circuit: Mix and match workouts from earlier in the week to create a demanding circuit.

Take a 15-second break after every 30 seconds of exercise.

Finish the circuit's five rounds.

Once you've reached Day 60, analyse your strength/endurance levels, measurements, and images to evaluate your improvement.

- **Monitor your progress with the tips given earlier**

Day 61-90: Advanced Workouts

- **Day 61-62**

Push-Ups: Perform 4 sets of 18–20 repetitions.

Bodyweight Squats: Perform four sets of 30 to 35 bodyweight squats.

Planks: Increase to four sets of 90–120 seconds for the planks.

Mountain Climbers: Aim for four sets of 35–40 repetitions per leg, mountain climbers.

- **Day 63-64**

Cardio workouts: Increase the duration of your cardio workout to 70–80 minutes.

HIIT Session: Set a higher bar for yourself by completing longer, high-intensity intervals, like 60 seconds of vigorous exercise and 45 seconds of restorative low-intensity activity.

- **Day 65-66**

Diamond Push-Ups: Perform 4 sets of 15–20 repetitions.

Tricep dips: 4 sets of 25–30 repetitions.

Russian twists: Increase to 4 sets of 30–35 repetitions per side for Russian twists.

Plank rotations: Attempt four sets of 25–30 repetitions per side for plank rotations.

- **Day 67-68**

Bodyweight Squats: Perform four sets of thirty to forty squats.

Lunges: Do 30 to 35 lunges per leg in four sets.

Glute Bridges on One Leg: Increase to Four Sets, 30–35 Reps Per Leg.

Calf Raises: Perform 4 sets of 30–35 repetitions.

- **Day 69-70**

Full Body Circuit: Mix and match workouts from earlier in the week to create a demanding circuit.

Take a 15-second break after every 30 seconds of exercise.

Finish the circuit's five rounds.

Once Day 70 has passed, analyse your strength/endurance levels, measurements, and images to determine how far you've come.

- **Day 71-72**

Push-Ups: Perform 4 sets of 18–20 repetitions.

Bodyweight squats: Perform four sets of 35–40 bodyweight squats.

Planks: Increase to four sets of 120–150 seconds for the planks.

Mountain Climbers:: Aim for four sets of forty to forty-five repetitions per leg.

- Day 73-74

Cardio workout: Increase the duration of your cardio workout to 80–90 minutes.

HIIT Session: Set a higher bar for yourself by completing longer, high-intensity intervals, like 60 seconds of vigorous exercise and 45 seconds of restorative low-intensity activity.

- Day 75-76

Diamond Push-Ups: Perform 4 sets of 18–20 repetitions.

Tricep dip: Do four sets of 30–35 repetitions for the tricep
dip.

Russian twists: Increase to 4 sets of 35–40 repetitions per side for Russian twists.

Plank Rotations: Try to complete 4 sets of 30–35 repetitions on each side.

- **Day 77-78**

Bodyweight squats: Perform four sets of 40–45 bodyweight squats.

Lunges: Do 35–40 lunges per leg in 4 sets.

Glute Bridges on One Leg: Increase to Four Sets, 35–40 Reps Per Leg.

Calf Raises: Perform 4 sets of 35–40 repetitions.

- **Day 79-80**

Full Body Circuit: Mix and match workouts from earlier in the week to create a demanding circuit.

Take a 15-second break after every 30 seconds of exercise.

Complete the circuit's six rounds.

Once Day 80 has passed, check your strength/endurance levels, measurements, and images to determine your progress and accomplishments.

- **Day 81-82**

Push-Ups: Perform 4 sets of 18–20 repetitions.

Bodyweight squats: Complete four sets of 40–45 bodyweight squats.

Planks: Increase to four sets of 150–180 seconds for the planks.

Mountain climbers: Aim for four sets of 45–50 repetitions per leg, mountain climbers.

- **Day 83-84**

Cardio workout: Increase the duration of your cardio workout to 90–100 minutes.

HIIT Session: Set a higher bar for yourself by completing longer, high-intensity intervals, like

60 seconds of vigorous exercise and 45 seconds of restorative low-intensity activity.

- **Day 85-86**

Diamond Push-Ups: Perform 4 sets of 20–22 repetitions.

Tricep Dips: 4 sets of 35–40 repetitions.

Russian twists: Increase to 4 sets of 40–45 repetitions per side for Russian twists.

Plank rotations: Try to complete 4 sets of 35–40 repetitions on each side.

- **Day 87-88**

Bodyweight squats: Perform four sets of 45–50 bodyweight squats.

Lunges: Do 40–45 lunges in 4 sets for each leg.

Glute Bridges on One Leg: Increase to Four Sets, 40–45 Reps Per Leg.

Calf Raises: Perform 4 sets of 40–45 repetitions.

- **Day 89-90**

Final Full Body Circuit: Mix and match exercises from earlier in the week to create a challenging circuit.

Take a 15-second break after every 30 seconds of exercise.

Complete the circuit's six rounds.

Celebrate your amazing accomplishments by conducting your final victory evaluation after Day 90 by looking over your measurements, pictures, and strength/endurance levels.

Celebrate Your Achievements

Full Body Workout Routines

- **Upper Body Exercises**

Including upper body workouts in your training is crucial to developing strength and a well-rounded, balanced body. These workouts focus on the arms, back, shoulders, and chest, among other upper body muscular areas. These are a few efficient upper body workouts:

1. Push-ups

Targets: Core, triceps, shoulders, and chest. How to: Spread your hands slightly wider than shoulder-width apart and begin in the plank posture. Once your chest is nearly touching the floor, bend your elbows to lower your body and then push yourself back up.

2. Pull-ups:

Targets: Shoulders, biceps, and back.

How to: Hang with your palms facing away from a pull-up bar. After raising your chin above the bar with your body, return to the lower position.

3. Bench Press with Dumbbell:

Targets: triceps, shoulders, and chest.
How to: Hold a dumbbell in each hand while lying on a bench. Dumbbells are raised by pressing, lowered to the chest, and then raised again.

4. Bent-Over Rows:

Targets: Biceps, lats, and upper back.
How to: Hold a barbell or dumbbells while bending at the hips. With your back straight, pull the weight to your waist.

5. Shoulder press with dumbbells:

Targets: Triceps and shoulders.

How to: Stand or sit on a bench with back support. Press each dumbbell overhead while holding it in each hand at shoulder height.

6. Bicep Curls:

Targets: Biceps.
How to: With your palms facing forward, hold a dumbbell in each hand. Curl the weights in the direction of your shoulders without moving your upper arms.

7. Tricep dips:

Targets: Shoulders and triceps
How to: Make use of a stable platform or parallel bars. Bend your elbows to lower your body, then push yourself back up.

8. Raises Raises:

Targets: Shoulders.

How to: Keep a dumbbell at your sides in each hand. Raise and then descend your arms to shoulder level.

9. Diamond Push-Ups:

Targets: Shoulders, chest, and triceps.
How to: Press your hands together beneath your chest to perform a push-up, making a diamond shape with your fingers.

10:Plank Rows

Targets: Shoulders, core, and back.
How to: Hold a dumbbell in each hand and begin in the plank position. Keeping your balance with the other arm, row one dumbbell to your hip and then swap sides.

To improve your total upper body fitness, strengthen your muscles, and boost their definition, incorporate these upper body workouts into your programme. Make sure you use the right form and technique, and as you gain strength, gradually challenge yourself by adding weight or reps.

- **Lower Body Exercises**

It is essential to strengthen your lower body for both general functional fitness and sports performance. These lower body workouts focus on the quadriceps, hamstrings, glutes, and calves, among other leg muscles. These are a few efficient lower body workouts:

1. Squats with bodyweight:

Target muscles: Hamstrings, glutes, calves, and quadriceps.
How to: Place your feet shoulder-width apart while standing. While maintaining a straight back, bend your knees and lower your body. Then, push through your heels to stand back up.

2. Squats:

Target muscles: Hamstrings, glutes, calves, and quadriceps.

How to: Take a single stride forward, then lower your body until your knees are 90 degrees bent. Go back to the beginning and alternate your legs.

3. Deadlifts:

Target muscles: lower back, glutes, hamstrings, and traps.
How to: Place dumbbells or a barbell in front of your thighs while standing with your feet hip-width apart. Lower the weight to the ground while maintaining a straight back at the hips, then stand back up.

4. Glutes Bridges:

Targetmuscles: lower back, hamstrings, and glutes.
How to: Place your feet flat on the floor and bend your knees while lying on your back. Squeeze your glutes to raise and then descend your hips off the ground.

5. Calf Raises:

Target Muscles: Heifers.
How to: Place your feet hip-width apart. Step up onto your toes and then step back down onto your heels.

6. Step-Ups:

Target muscles: glutes, hamstrings, and quadriceps.
How to: Place one foot on a platform or bench and raise the other one. Resuming with the opposite leg, step back down.

7. Squats in Bulgarian Split:

Target muscles: glutes, hamstrings, and quadriceps.
How to: Step one foot on the bench behind you, step forward a few steps in front of it, and drop your body into a lunge. Change your legs and go back to the beginning position.

8. Leg Press:

Target muscles: glutes, hamstrings, and quadriceps.
How to: While seated on a leg press machine, extend your legs by pressing the weighted platform away from you.

9. Wall-Sits:

Target muscles: Glute and quadriceps.
How to: Slid down till your thighs are parallel to the floor while leaning your back against the wall. Hold the position.

10. Sumo Squat

Target muscles The quadriceps, hamstrings, glutes, and inner thighs are the targets.
How to: Position your feet wider than shoulder-width apart, with your toes pointing outward. After lowering yourself into a squat, raise yourself back up.

To increase your lower body fitness, strengthen your lower body, and improve your stability, incorporate these exercises into your workout regimen. As you advance, you can challenge your muscles even more by increasing the weights or repetitions, but proper form and technique are still crucial.

- **Core Strengthening Workouts**

The basis for total strength, stability, and balance is a robust core. Exercises that strengthen your core focus on the muscles in your lower back, pelvis, and abdomen. These workouts strengthen your spine, help you develop a toned core, and enhance your general athletic performance. These are a few efficient exercises for strengthening the core:

1.Planks:

Targets: Lower back, obliques, and the entire core.
How to: Place your forearms on the ground to start in the push-up posture. For as long as you

can, maintain a straight body, contract your core, and hold the pose.

2. Russian Twists:

Targets: the lower back, rectus abdominis (front abs), and obliques.
How to: Take a seat on the floor with your feet off the ground and your knees bent. Take a little step back and rotate your body such that both hands contact the ground on either side.

3. Bicycle crunchies:

Targets: Transverse abdominis, rectus abdominis, and obliques.
How to : Place your hands behind your head while lying on your back. Raise your arms over your head, shoulders, and legs, then switch between bringing your right elbow to your left knee and your left knee to your right.

4. Leg Raises:

Targets: Lower back.
How to: Prop your legs straight while lying on your back. Straightening your legs as you lift them off the ground, bring them back down without making contact with the ground.

5. Mountain climbers:

Targets: Shoulders, hip flexors, and core.
How to: Start by assuming a plank posture. Keeping the opposite leg extended, bring one knee up to the chest. When running, switch up your leg movements.

6. Hollow Body Hold:

Targets: Lower back and whole core.
How to: Extend your arms and legs off the ground while lying on your back. Maintaining your lower back pressed into the floor, raise your head, shoulders and feet just a little bit off the ground.

7. Hanging Leg Raises

Targets: Hip flexors, lower back, and lower abs.
How to: Raise your legs straight out in front of
you while hanging from a pull-up bar, then
lower them back down.

8. Side Planks:

Targets: Lateral core muscles and obliques.
How to: Assume a side laying position, placing
your elbow just beneath your shoulder. Raise
your hips off the floor so that your head and
heels are in a straight line.

9. L-Sits:

Targets: entire core, encompassing the hip
flexors and abs.
How to: Take a seat on the floor and extend your
legs in front of you. With your hands on the
floor next to your hips, raise your body off the
ground so that your legs and torso form an L.

10. Swiss Ball Rollouts

Targets: Lower back, obliques, and the entire core.
How to: Roll a Swiss ball forward as far as you can while maintaining an engaged core while kneeling in front of it and placing your forearms on it. Roll it back to where you started.

To develop a strong and stable core, incorporate these exercises into your training regimen. In addition to improving your physical performance, having a strong core also helps you to

Conclusion

Well done on finishing your 90-day fitness challenge! It's amazing that you've committed time and energy to enhancing your health and wellbeing. We really hope that this book, the "90 Day No Equipment Workout Plan," will be a helpful guide for you as you embark on a more active and healthy lifestyle.

You've learned throughout the course of these ninety-nine days the value of perseverance, consistency, and the health benefits of physical and mental fitness. You've pushed boundaries, conquered obstacles, and revelled in your accomplishments. You've made progress towards becoming a better and healthier version of yourself thanks to your dedication to this adventure.

Recall that this is only the beginning of your fitness journey as you end this chapter. The routines and information you've acquired will act as a cornerstone for your continued dedication to fitness and wellness. Keep establishing new objectives, looking for novel challenges, and investigating various facets of wellness.

We want to sincerely thank you for selecting this book, for making a health investment, and for making positive changes in your life. We appreciate your participation in this journey and letting us share in your success in being fit.

Continue being a cheerful, energetic person who always aspires to be the greatest version of herself. You should put your all into maintaining and improving your health and well-being. Even though there is still more to go, keep in mind that you are already a fitness champion. Continue on your route, and may it be paved with resilience, vigour, and all the benefits that come with leading a healthier lifestyle.

I appreciate you and wish you a happier, better, and busier future.

www.ingramcontent.com/pod-product-compliance
Lightning Source LLC
Chambersburg PA
CBHW070822280726

48660CB00017B/2647